Understanding Deep Vein Thrombosis

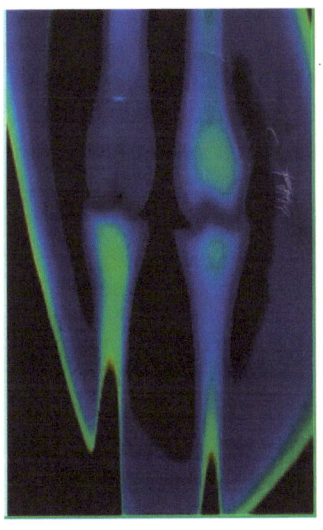

Written and Published by
Claudia Barros MSN RN CCM
7821 North 173rd Avenue
Waddell AZ 85355

For my husband, T.C.

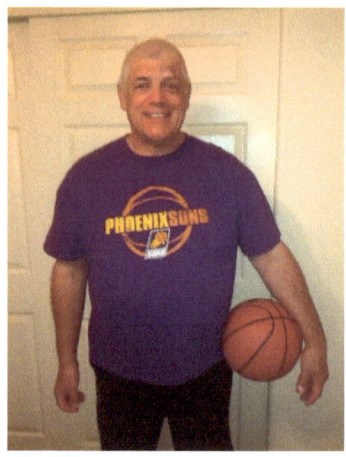

Blood Clot Basics

DVTs are blood clots (thrombosis) within the large deep veins of the legs or arms. The deep veins are responsible for transporting over 90% of the blood returned to the heart.

These blood clots can be caused by injury, trauma, inflammation, or disease. The injured lining of the vein causes blood flow to be slowed, platelets to collect, fibrin to form, and clots to develop.

These clots can be temporary or permanent, partially or completely block-ing the blood flow within the vein. The blockage causes the vein to become dilated and the pressure within the vessel to increase.

Permanent damage to the valves and the surrounding tissue can occur as a result of the increased pressure, stretching, oxygen deprivation and lack of nutrients.

The mechanism that allows for normal fluid and electrolyte exchange between the capillaries and surrounding tissue can be affected. Damaged capillaries may function normally when the person is lying down while showing inadequate fluid exchange when standing or sitting.

Blood clots cause varying degrees of obstruction to blood flow depending on the size and location of the vein involved. If the clot occurs in a small vein, collateral circulation will compensate. This may also be true if the clotting occurs in the deep veins of the leg or in a larger vein of the arm. Collateral channels may develop even after obstruction of the superior or inferior vena cava.

When a blood clot occurs in a large, deep vein, the collateral circulation will compensate only partially. This causes the pressure in the vein to increase beyond the site of the clot. This increased pressure results in distention of all veins in the limb and causes intense congestion of the area. Swelling (edema) of the affected limb then develops.

Small clots (emboli) may dislodge from the larger clot and travel through the blood stream. These clots can be life threatening if they are large enough and become lodged in the heart, lungs or brain. The most common clots are those that travel to the lungs (pulmonary emboli).

Over time, even after a blood clot has been reabsorbed, obstruction of the vein may continue to occur. This is due to the remaining fibrous tissue bands left behind by the chronic damage.

DVTs can also occur without symptoms.

Vein, Valves & Blood Flow

In the lower extremity the three groups of veins — deep, communicating and superficial — normally have thin elastic walls and valves that function like gates. The action of the calf muscle and the properly functioning valves allow blood to flow against gravity on its way back to the heart. Muscular compression of the elastic veins forces the blood upward and the valves prevent back flow.

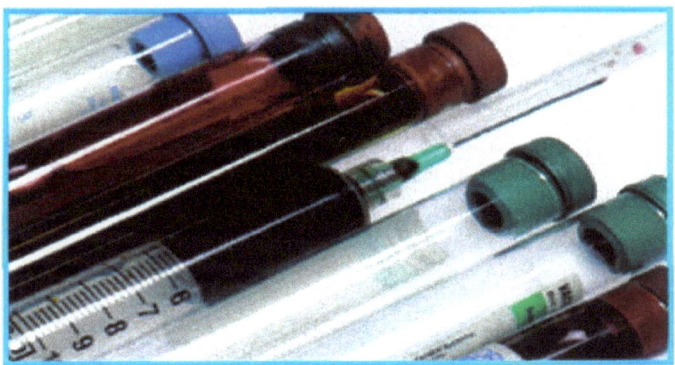

Failure of Normal Mechanism

The normal mechanism of the veins and valves fails when chronic DVTs are present, usually because of extensive damage to vessel walls and valves. Damage results from the slowing of venous blood flow within the partially or completely obstructed vessels. Vessel walls become thickened and inelastic while the damaged valves stop functioning properly.

With prolonged standing, the venous pressure increases dramatically, and this upsets the normal equilibrium of capillary fluid exchange. Blood flow is slowed and congestion and swelling develop.

Sedentary Lifestyle

Immobility and prolonged sitting contribute to poor circulation and clot development. This is due to the slowing of the blood flow.

The primary causes of immobility are surgical procedures lasting longer than one hour and illness or injury that results in prolonged bedrest or loss of use of the injured extremity.

A sedentary lifestyle slows blood flow in the legs, reducing circulation and increasing the risk for blood clot formation. This is why it is so important to stay active as you get older.

Regular walking is the best activity for improving blood flow in the legs.

The Skin & Tissue

In the leg and ankle, below the level of the clot, changes can occur to the skin and tissue. These changes include swelling, warmth over the area, (blue, red or orange) discoloration, irritation, and ulcers.

The veins under the skin may become dilated and more or less visible depending upon where the swelling occurs.

Fever and chills may occur. Muscle cramps are common.

An intense burning sensation occurs when the swelling and fluid stasis put pressure on the nerves in the affected limb. This burning sensation tends to subside after the excess fluid drains from the arm or leg.

Pain may or may not be present. It is usually described as more severe when standing rather than walking. A dull ache or deep soreness develops in the affected leg after standing or sitting for extended periods of time.

The pain usually disappears within 10-30 minutes after assuming a lying down position and elevating the leg, except when the swelling has become excessive.

To prevent tissue damage, you should avoid extensive swelling. Balance the benefits of moderate activity by including periods of rest with elevation of the affected limb above the level of the heart.

Conventional Medicine

Hospitalization & Heparin therapy — The initial treatment for DVTs is intravenous heparin therapy, regulated by PTT testing. Hospital care also includes: bedrest, moderate activity, warm moist heat and elevation of the affected limb.

Coumadin therapy — Long term DVT therapy often consists of oral doses of coumadin (warfarin sodium) monitored regularly by PT/INR testing.

Aspirin — some studies show that low dose aspirin (less than one regular tablet per day) may be as effective as stronger anticoagulants in treating DVTs.

New Drugs — can also be used as alternatives to Coumadin therapy, they include Eliquis (Apixaban), Pradaxa (Dabigatran), Savaysa (Edoxaban), and Xarelto (Rivaroxaban).

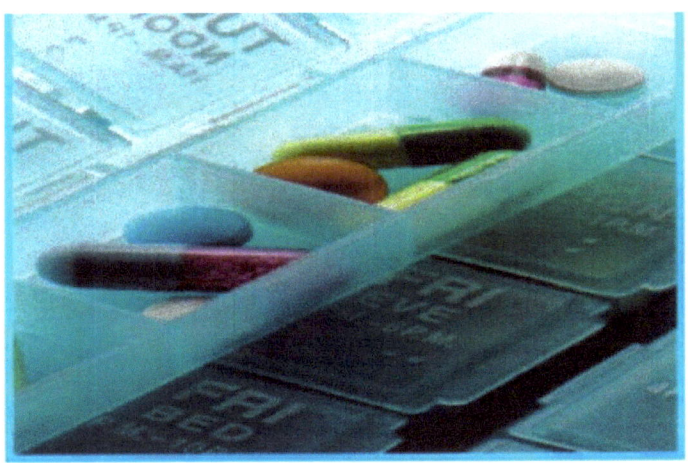

Vitamins & Minerals

Magnesium plus Calcium — A natural blood thinner that reduces abnormal clotting.

Vitamin C with bioflavonoids — Aids circulation and reduces clotting tendencies.

Vitamin B6, B3, Lipotrophic, Bromelain, Manganese — Are needed to assimilate calcium, iron & vitamins. They help reduce stress and promote healing of damaged tissue.

Vitamin E with Zinc — Thins the blood and reduces platelet stickiness.

Take a complete vitamin & mineral supplement, containing 100% of the Recommended Daily Allowances.

If taking Coumadin regularly, find a vitamin supplement that does not include Vitamin K. Vitamin K naturally makes the blood clot more easily.

Herbal Remedies & Macronutrients

Omega-3 & Omega-6 Fatty acids — Fish benefits the heart by making blood less prone to abnormal clotting. The Omega-3 & Omega-6 fats in fish are credited with this effect. Consume cold water fish three times per week.

Garlic — Large amounts of garlic (10-12 cloves per day) enhance the process by which our bodies break up potentially dangerous blood clots. The active ingredient in garlic resides in the oil, which is unstable, therefore garlic should be used in its fresh form and not in capsules.

Garlic goes wonderfully with sauteed foods, in slow cooked meals such as stews, roasted, or in vinegar and oil dressings.

Onions — Onions appear to have the same beneficial effects against abnormal blood clots as garlic. They can be used raw, roasted, stewed or sauteed. Blanch whole onions, then peel, stuff and bake.

Use sautéed onions on top of pizza or pasta. Add raw onions to oil and vinegar dressing over salad greens.

Flaxseed oil — Supplies essential fatty acids in order to keep veins pliable and soft. This reduces the chance of blood clot formation.

Grape seed extract — Antioxidant that restores flexibility to vessel walls and reduces the risk of clot formation.

Alfalfa, Pau d'arco, Red raspberry, Rosemary, Yarrow — Antioxidants which improve blood oxygenation.

Cayenne — Thins the blood and improves circulation.

Butcher's broom, Skullcap, Valerian root, Ginkgo biloba, Hawthorne berry — Dilates blood vessels and improves circulation. Ginkgo has antioxidant effects.

Motherwort, Myrrh & Tumeric — Helps prevent the formation of blood clots.

Ginger — Can help prevent blood clots that trigger heart attacks and strokes. Eat gingerbread and drink ginger ale or ginger tea.

Ginseng — Has an anti-clotting (anti-platelet) effect, which helps reduce the risk of forming clots. Use root powder, teas, capsules or tablets.

Meadowsweet — May help prevent blood clot formation in the same manner as aspirin. As a tea, drink up to 3 cups per day. In a tincture, take 1/2 to 1 teaspoon up to 3 times a day.

Lycium — Chinese herbal remedy that improves circulation of blood and increases the absorption of nutrients by the cells.

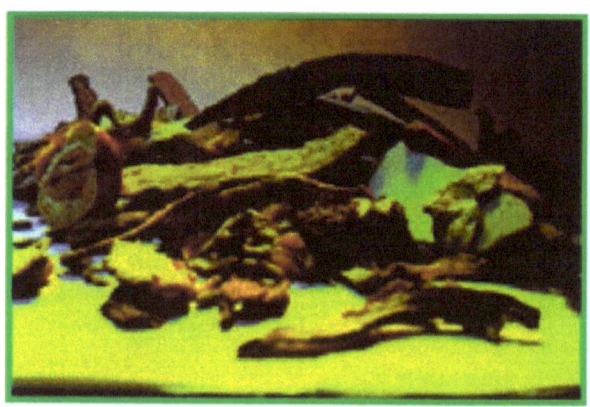

External Remedies

Warm Poultice — Applied directly to the affected area. Combine cayenne, ginger, plantain & witch hazel.

Care of leg ulcer — Use alcohol free goldenseal extract. Apply a dropperful of extract on a sterile piece of gauze and place over the affected area.

Elevation of Extremity — Raise the affected extremity above the level of the heart in order to promote the return of blood, improve circulation, reduce swelling, and relieve congestion.

Heat Applications — Use warm baths, heating pads, and warm whirlpool soaks to help promote the circulation of fluid back to the heart. This will keep your blood flowing freely and help prevent blood clot formation in the affected limb.

Nutrition

Eat plenty of fresh fruits and vegetables.

Consume raw nuts and seeds, soybean products, and whole grains.

Reduce or eliminate the consumption of red meat.

Do not consume dairy products, fried or salty foods, or partially hydrogenated vegetable oils.

Decrease sugar intake as sucrose increases platelet stickiness and clotting.

Fast periodically to rid the body of toxins.

Use Juice Therapy — garlic, carrot, parsley, spinach, celery & beets.

Green Leafy Vegetables

When taking Coumadin regularly, you can eat green leafy vegetables every day. However, it is important to eat approximately the same amount of leafy greens each day to maintain a constant intake of Vitamin K.

By balancing a constant and appropriate dose of Coumadin with the same amount of leafy green vegetables every day, you will maintaining a proper INR level.

In contrast, with many of the newer drugs used as alternatives to Coumadin therapy, your consumption of green leafy vegetables can vary greatly from day-to-day. This is because Vitamin K intake does not affect the anti-clotting mechanism of these newer drugs.

Vitamin K is the antidote for an overdose of Coumadin. Many of the newer drugs do not have an antidote for overdose. This is because they use an alternative mechanism unrelated to Vitamin K to promote the anti-clotting effect.

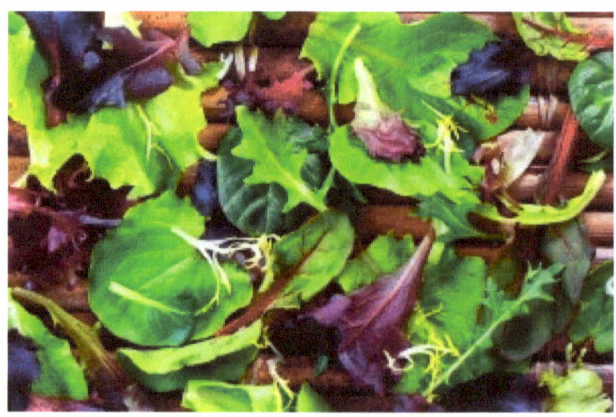

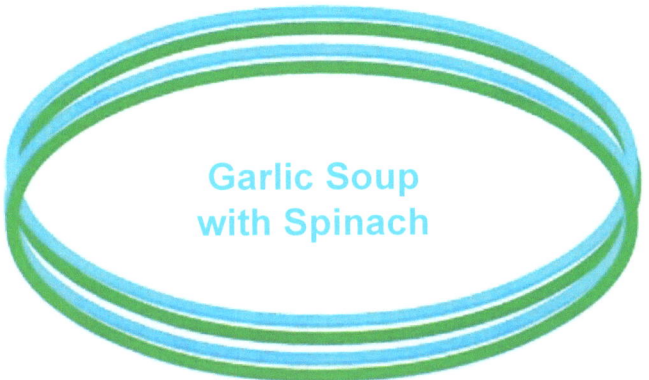

Garlic Soup
with Spinach

Ingredients for Soup

1 tablespoon olive oil
1 bulb garlic, peeled and separated into cloves
2 onions, chopped
3 bay leaves
1 teaspoon dried thyme
2 allspice berries, crushed
2 cups vegetable, chicken or beef stock
1 cup skim milk
1 large bunch of shredded fresh spinach

In a large stockpot, warm oil over medium heat. Add garlic, onions, bay leaves, thyme, allspice, and stock. Bring to a boil. Reduce heat and simmer until garlic is tender, about 15 minutes.

Discard bay leaves, then use slotted spoon to transfer garlic and onions to a food processor or blender. Add a splash of stock from the large stockpot, then process until smooth.

Add the garlic mixture from the food processor or blender back into the large stockpot and heat over low heat while adding milk. Continue to heat gently and stir until the soup is hot. Add spinach, stir briefly, then serve. (The hot soup will blanch the spinach perfectly.)

To remove the odor of garlic from your breath, chew a fresh sprig of parsley. To remove the aroma from your hands, use toothpaste and rinse.

Exercise

Get regular moderate exercise 30 to 60 minutes every day.

Walking, swimming, jogging, playing tennis, bike riding, shooting baskets or walking your dog improves circulation, prevents sluggishness in the veins, and lessens the tendency to form clots.

> - Take a walk after dinner.
> - Sign-up for an exercise class.
> - Get off the bus one stop early and walk in a safe area.
> - Park your car farther away from the entrances to malls or stores.
> - Take the stairs instead of the elevator … one flight up or two flights down.

It is vital to stay active as you get older. This will help prevent the formation of DVTs.

Life Style Modifications

Avoid prolonged sitting on long airline flights or automobile trips, especially in cramped conditions.

Practical preventive measures for travelers:

> ➢ Get up and walk the aisle every hour.
> ➢ Stop at rest areas periodically.
> ➢ Wear loose and comfortable clothes.
> ➢ Frequently stretch your legs and pump your calf muscles by pointing your toes.
> ➢ Occasionally take deep breaths to help improve oxygenation to your body and legs.

Avoid wearing tight fitting clothes that cut off circulation — especially knee socks with tight bands.

Use special elastic support stockings (antiembolism stockings) to improve circulation when standing or sitting for any prolonged period.

Take hot baths and whirlpools daily. This helps promote circulation.

Lie down with your feet elevated above the level of your heart whenever possible. Take naps and rest breaks throughout the day and get at least 8 hours of sleep each night. When in bed, move your legs frequently to promote circulation and prevent the blood from pooling.

Prevent leg ulcers by keeping the skin clean. Avoid products that dry the skin. Redness and swelling may be signs of infection. If you develop leg ulcers, keep them clean and germ-free to prevent infection. Ulcers may take 3 months to 1 year to fully heal.

If you smoke, stop.

Notes: